50 Amazing Facts About Social Life

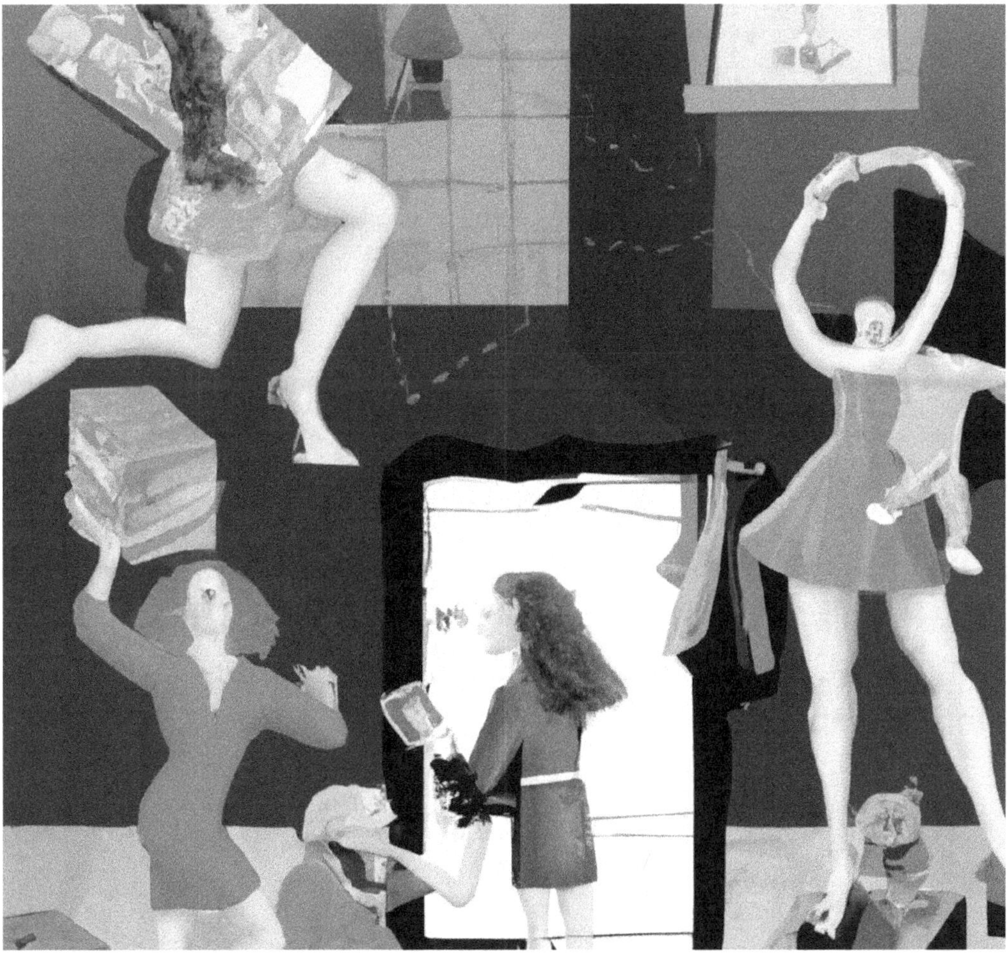

TABLE OF CONTENT

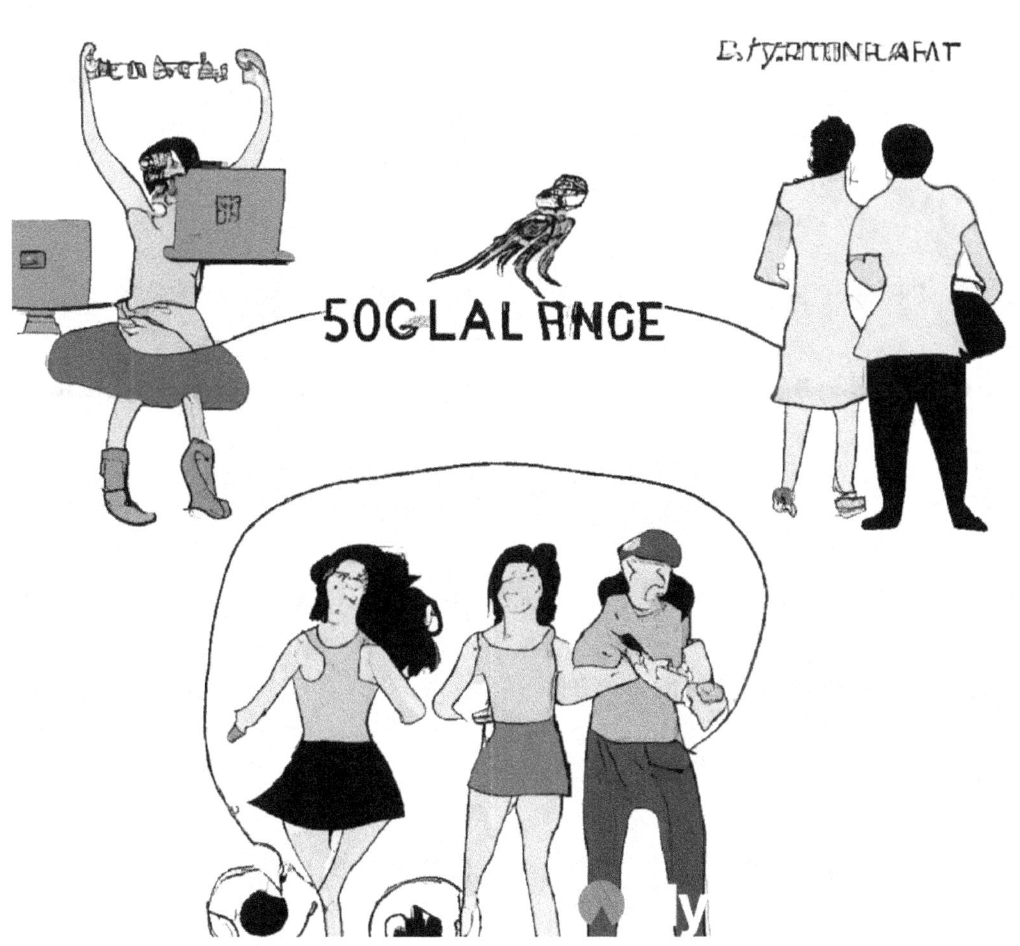
SOGLAL ANCE

Introduction

Whether you're single or in a relationship, there's always something new to learn about social life.

For instance, did you know that in some cultures, it's considered impolite to refuse a drink? Or that in ancient Greece, it was considered bad luck to meet a black cat?

In this post, we've gathered 50 amazing facts about social life that will surprise and fascinate you. From social customs to dating tips, we've got you covered. So sit back and get ready to learn something new!

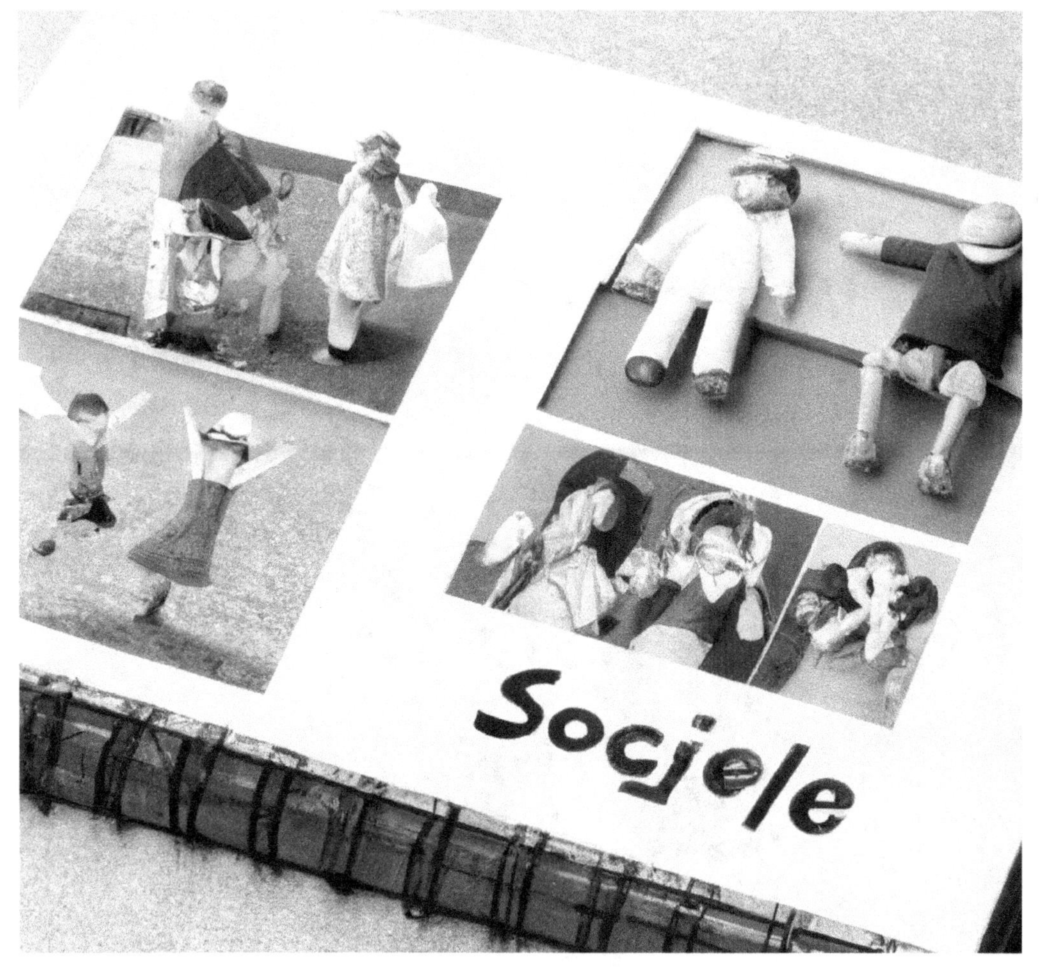

Socjele

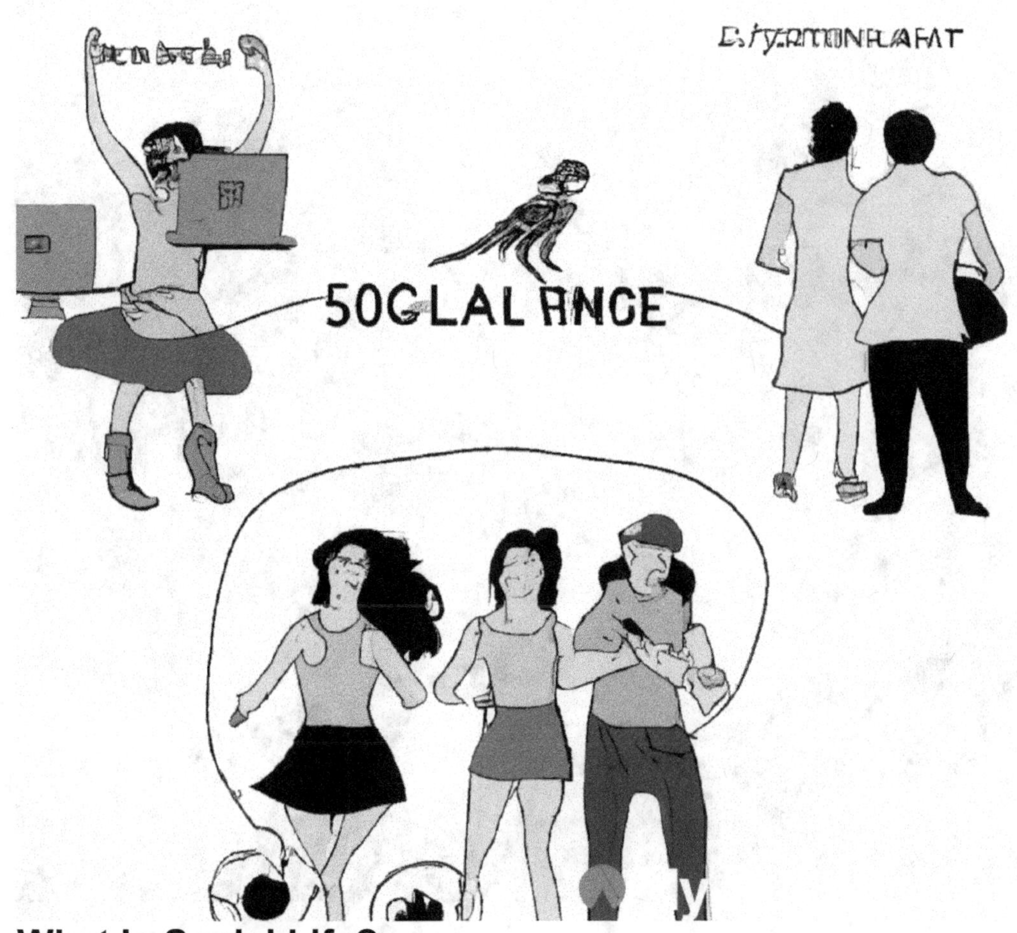

What Is Social Life?

What is social life? You might be thinking, "Isn't that just another way of saying 'social media'?" And while social media is a big part of social life, it's not the only thing.

In its simplest form, social life is the interaction we have with other people. It's the way we communicate, share our thoughts and feelings, and build relationships. Social life doesn't happen in a vacuum—it happens in the real world, with real people.

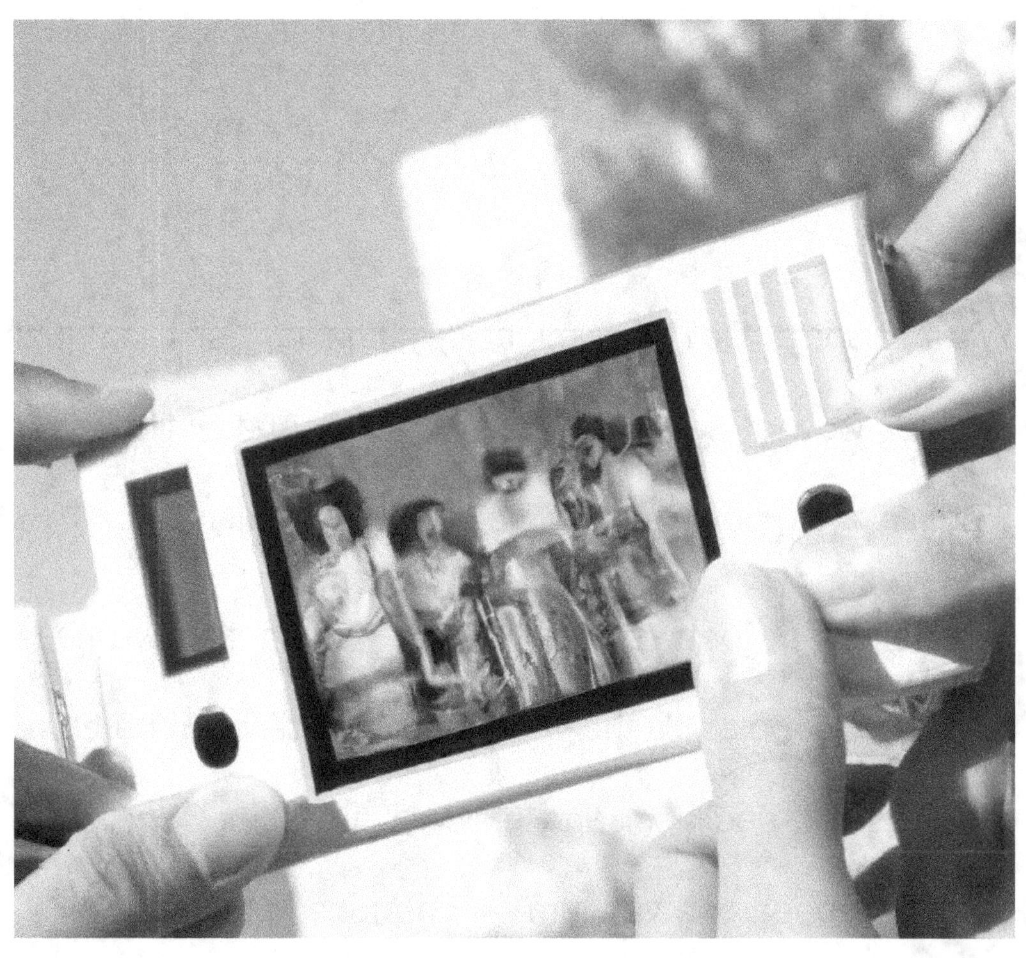

And that's what makes it so special. Social media can be great for staying in touch with friends and family, but there's nothing quite like sitting down face-to-face and having a conversation.

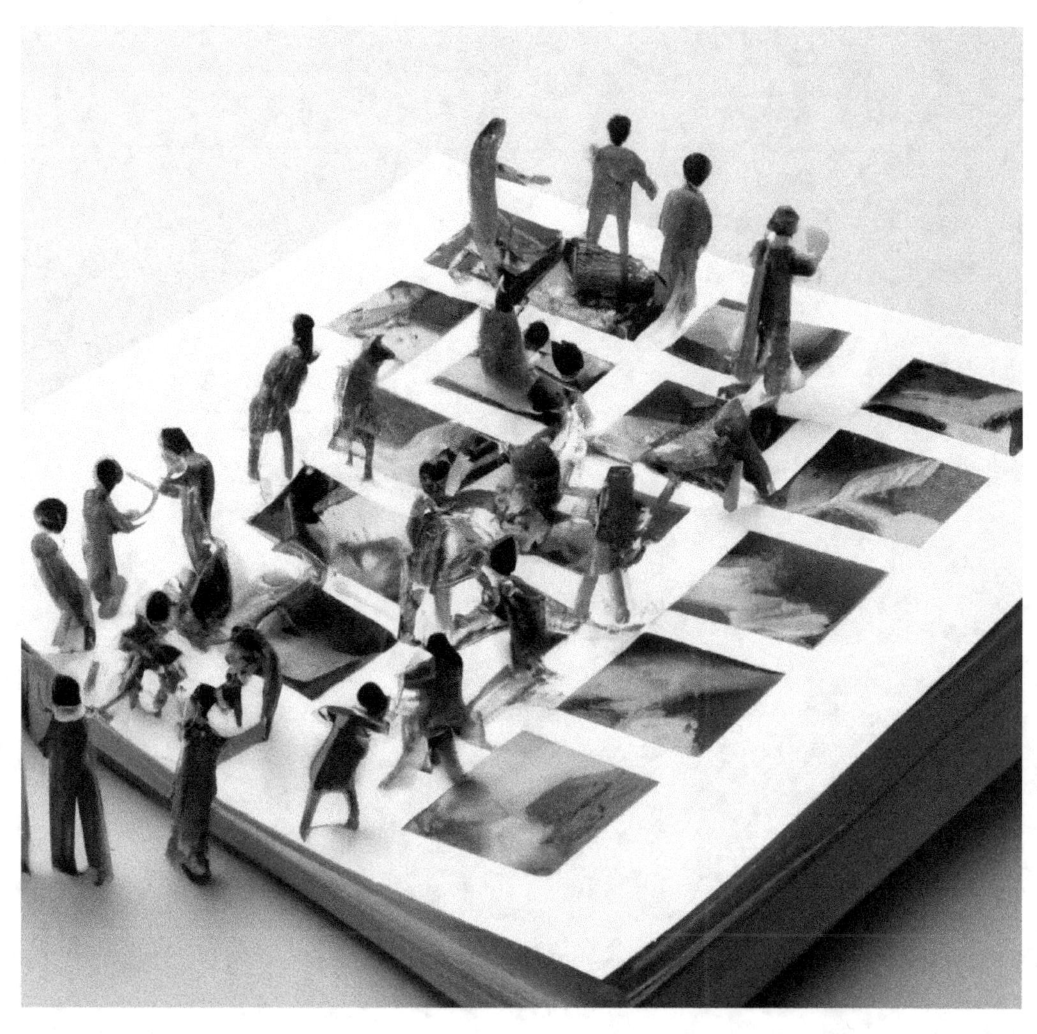

What Are the Benefits of Social Life?

Imagine living without social life. It would be quite boring, wouldn't it?

Humans are social animals, and we need interaction with others in order to feel happy and fulfilled. That's why social life is so important—it gives us the chance to connect with other people, share experiences, and have fun.

There are all sorts of benefits to socializing, from boosting our mood to helping us live longer. Here are just a few:

• Socializing makes us happy. Numerous studies have shown that people who have strong social networks are happier than those who don't. Human brains are hardwired for social interaction, and it feels good when we connect with others.

• Socializing makes us smarter. Research has shown that socializing helps keep our brains sharp as we age.

interacting with others helps us learn new things and keeps our minds active.

• Socializing makes us healthier. Studies have shown that those who have a strong social network tend to be healthier overall than those who don't. interacting with others helps us stay in shape, lowers our stress levels, and can even help fight off disease.

How Can Social Life Improve Your Mental Health?

You might not realize it, but your social life can have a significant impact on your mental health. Socializing with others is essential for our overall well-being, and it can help improve our moods, make us feel more connected, and even boost our self-esteem.

But of course, not all socializing is created equal. It's important to choose activities and friends that make you

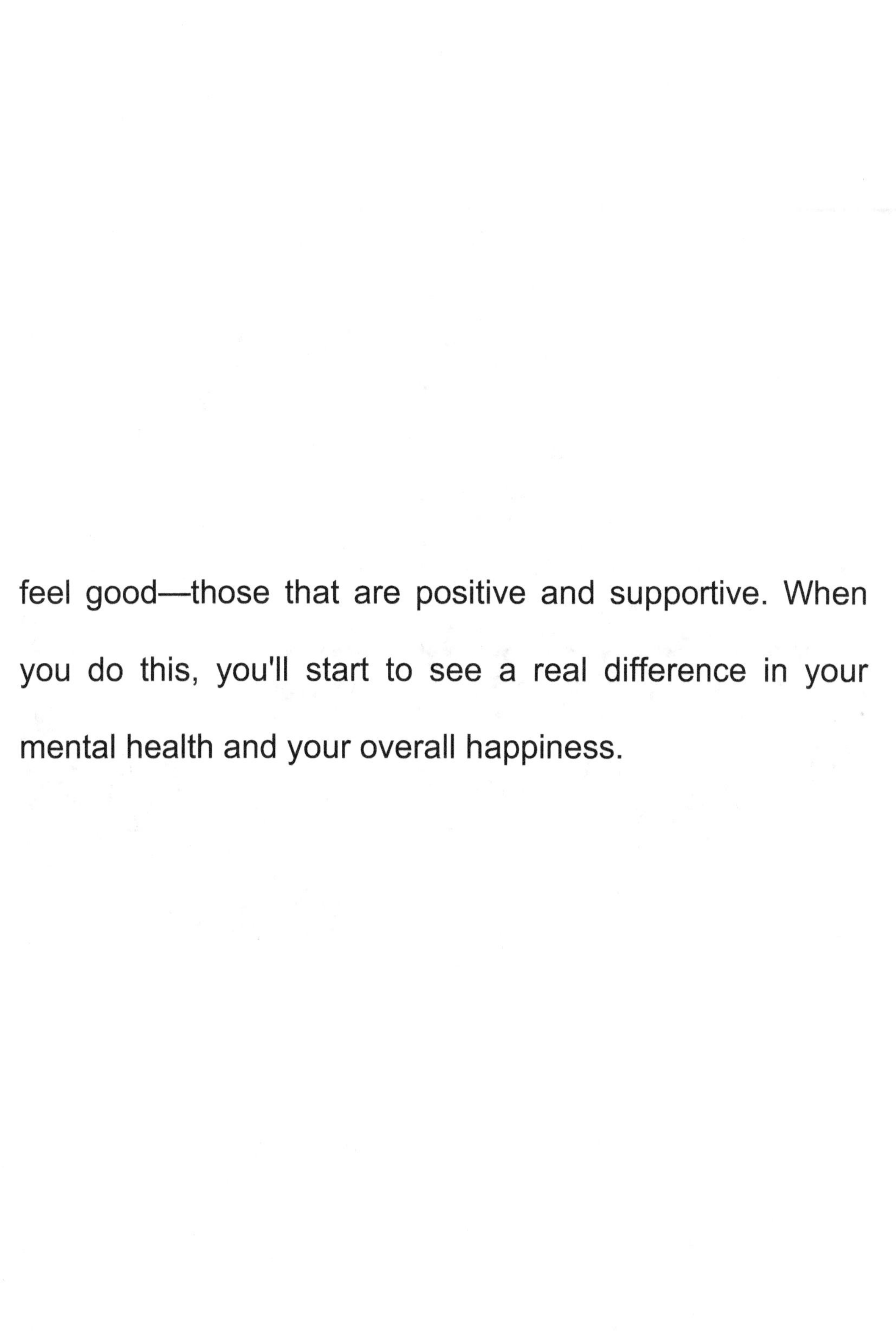

feel good—those that are positive and supportive. When you do this, you'll start to see a real difference in your mental health and your overall happiness.

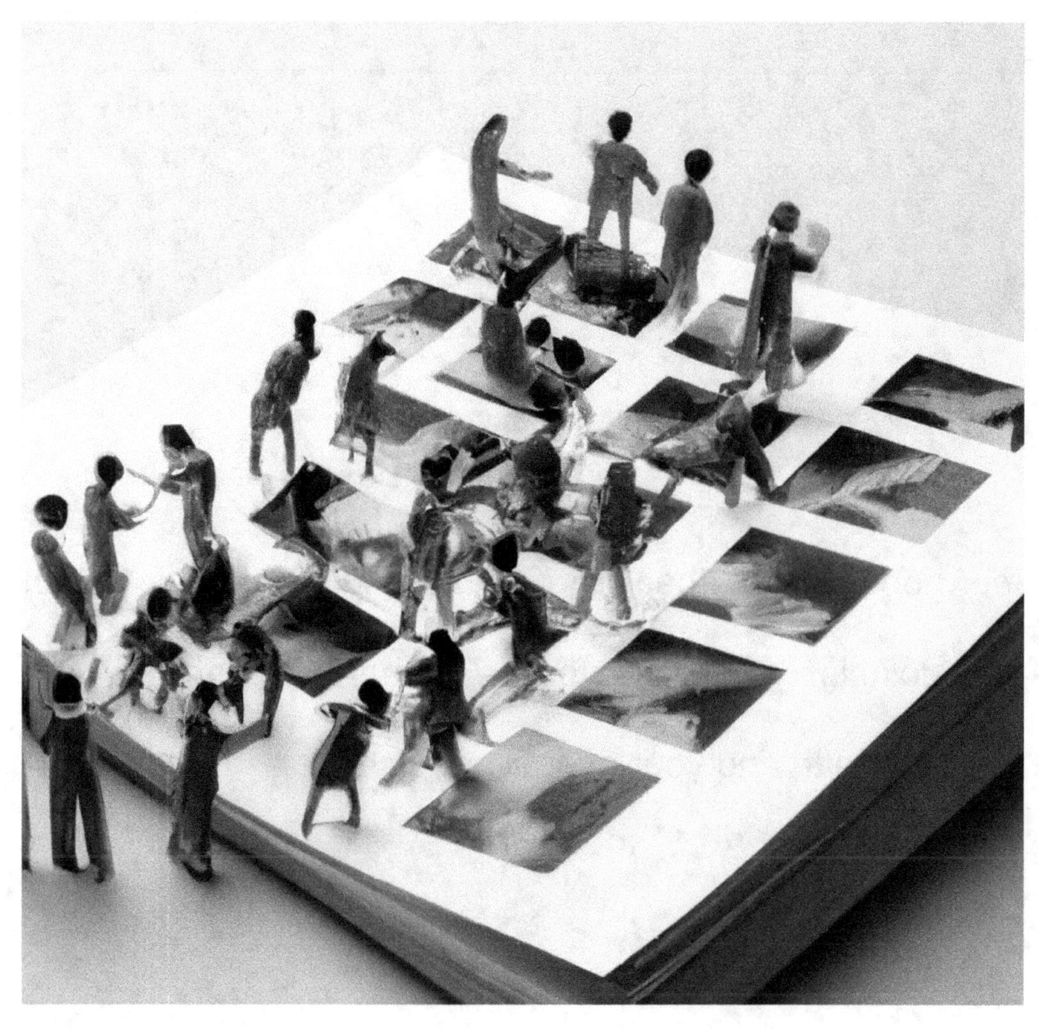

What Are the Best Ways to Meet New People and Make Friends?

So you're new in town and you want to meet people. What are the best ways to make friends? Well, here are a few ideas to get you started:

1. Join a club or sports team. When you're part of a group, it's easy to make friends because you have something in common.

2. Go to social events. Meetup.com is a great website for finding social events in your area.

3. Try out a new activity. Taking a dance class or learning how to play the guitar are great ways to meet new people and make friends.

4. Join an online forum or social networking site. This is a great way to meet people who share your interests.

5. Get involved in your community. Volunteering is a great way to meet people who share your values and make friends in the process

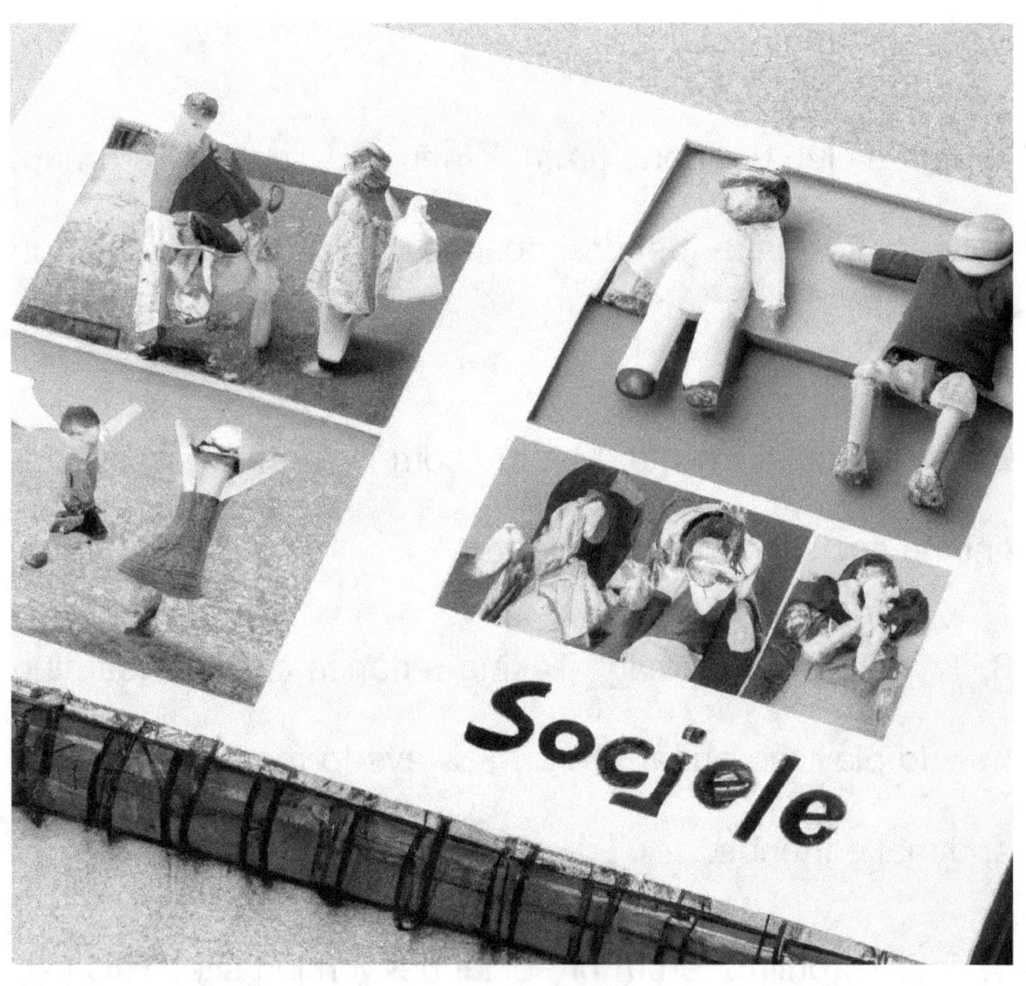

How Can Social Life Help You Overcome Anxiety and Depression?

Here's a thought for you: social life can help you overcome anxiety and depression. It sounds crazy, but it's true.

Social life is a great way to connect with other people and build meaningful relationships. When you're feeling down, it can be really helpful to talk to someone who will listen and understand.

And when you're feeling anxious, getting out there and meeting new people can actually help you calm down. It's all about interacting with the world in a positive way, which is the best way to fight off those negative feelings.

So go out there and enjoy social life! You'll be amazed at how much better you'll feel.

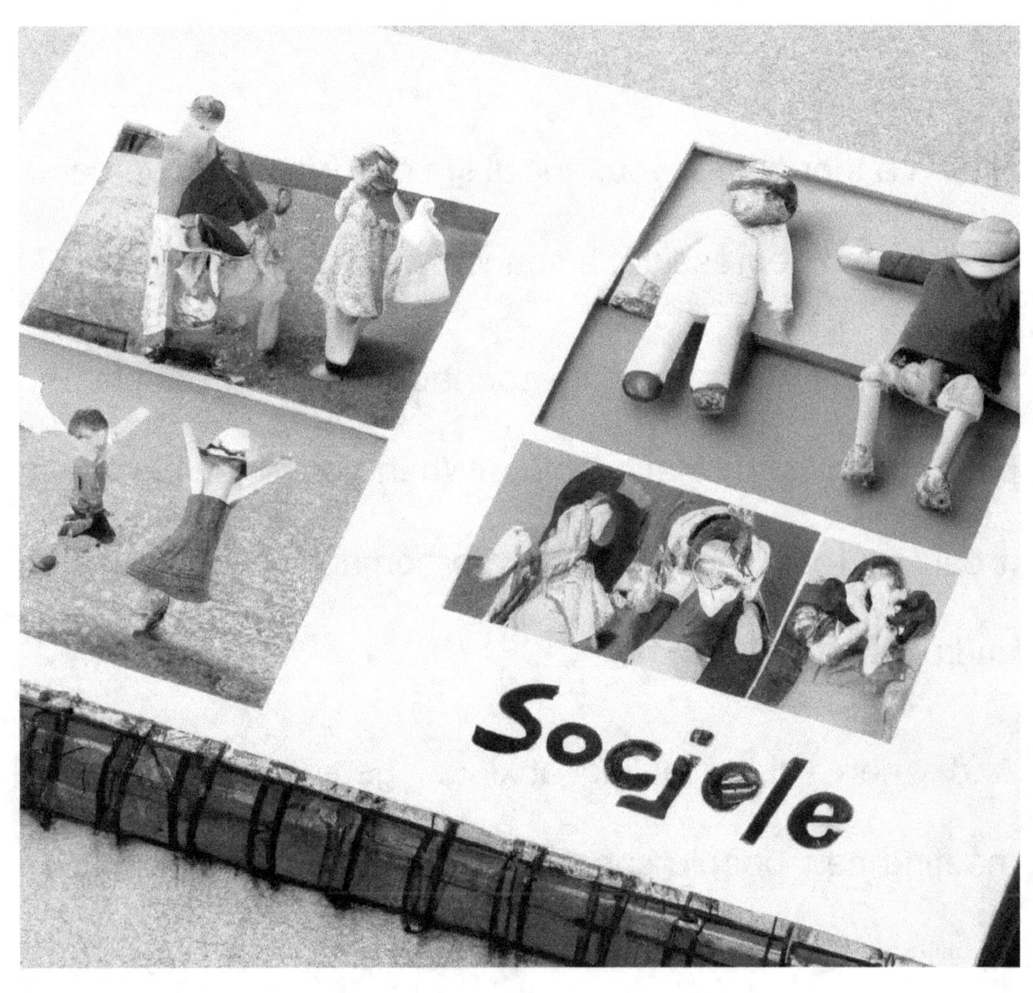

What Are the Best Ways to Stay Connected With Old Friends?

Keeping in touch with old friends can be a challenge, but it's definitely worth it.

Sometimes it feels like we're all so busy with our own lives that we don't have time for anything else. But if you really want to stay connected with your old friends, you'll find a way to make time. Here are some ideas:

1. Use social media to keep in touch. This is probably the easiest way to stay connected, and it's a great way to share updates about your life.

2. Meet up for coffee or lunch. This is a great way to catch up in person.

3. Schedule regular Skype dates. This is especially good if you live far away from your friends.

4. Organize a reunion party. This is a great way to celebrate your friendships!

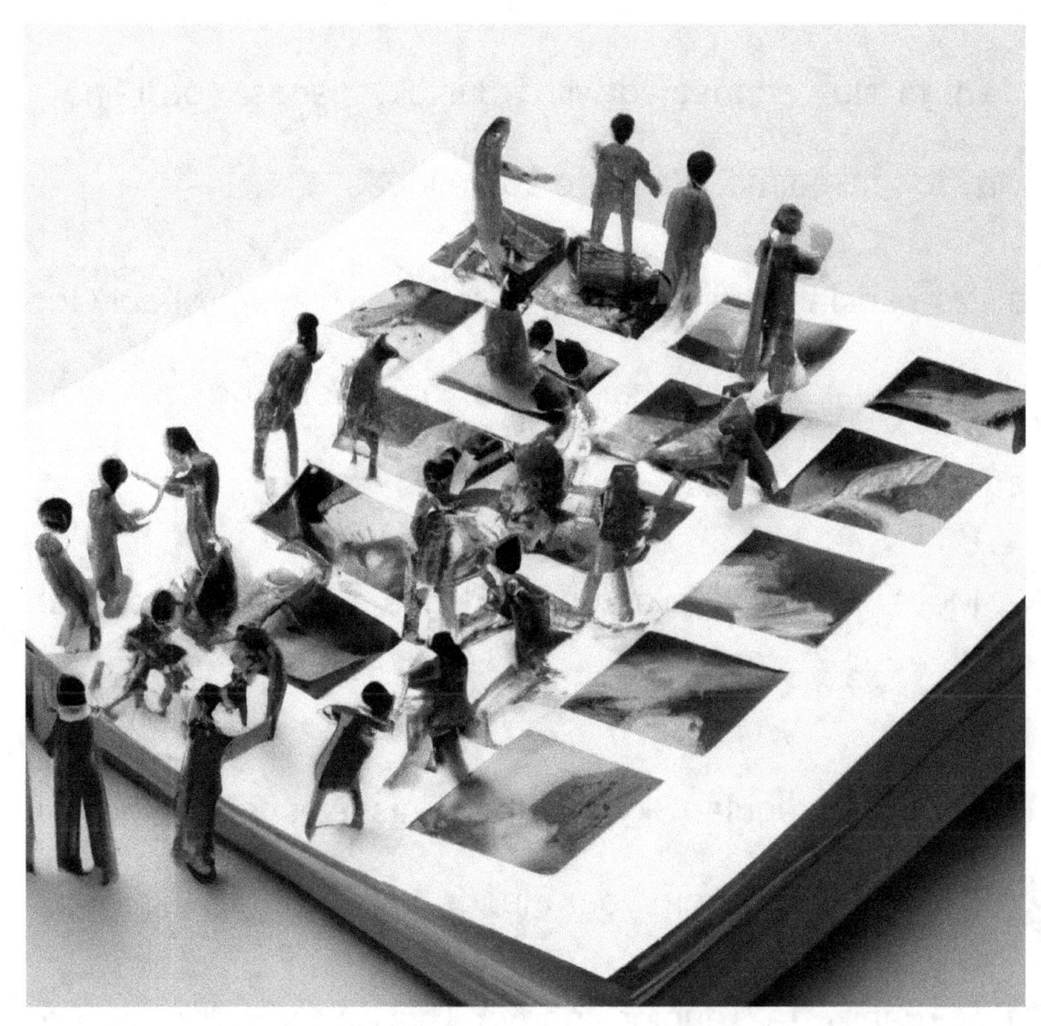

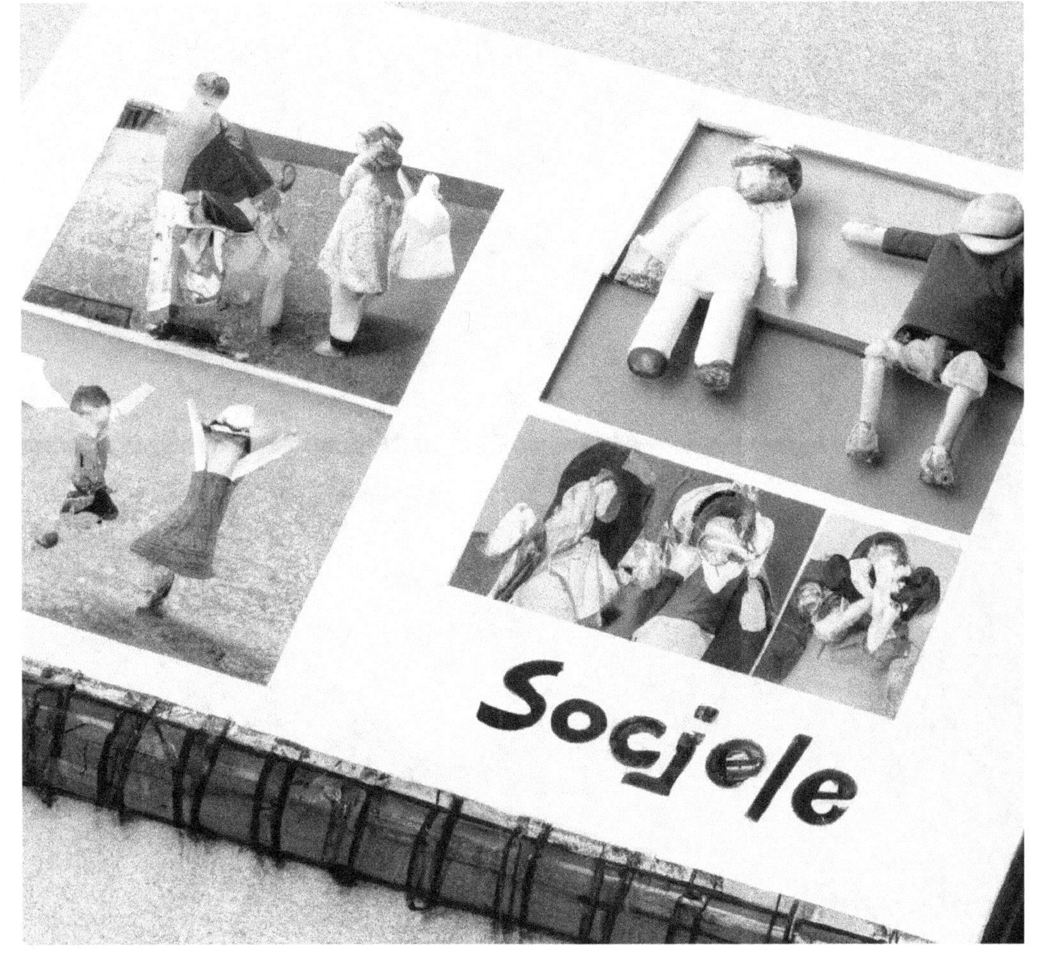
Sociele

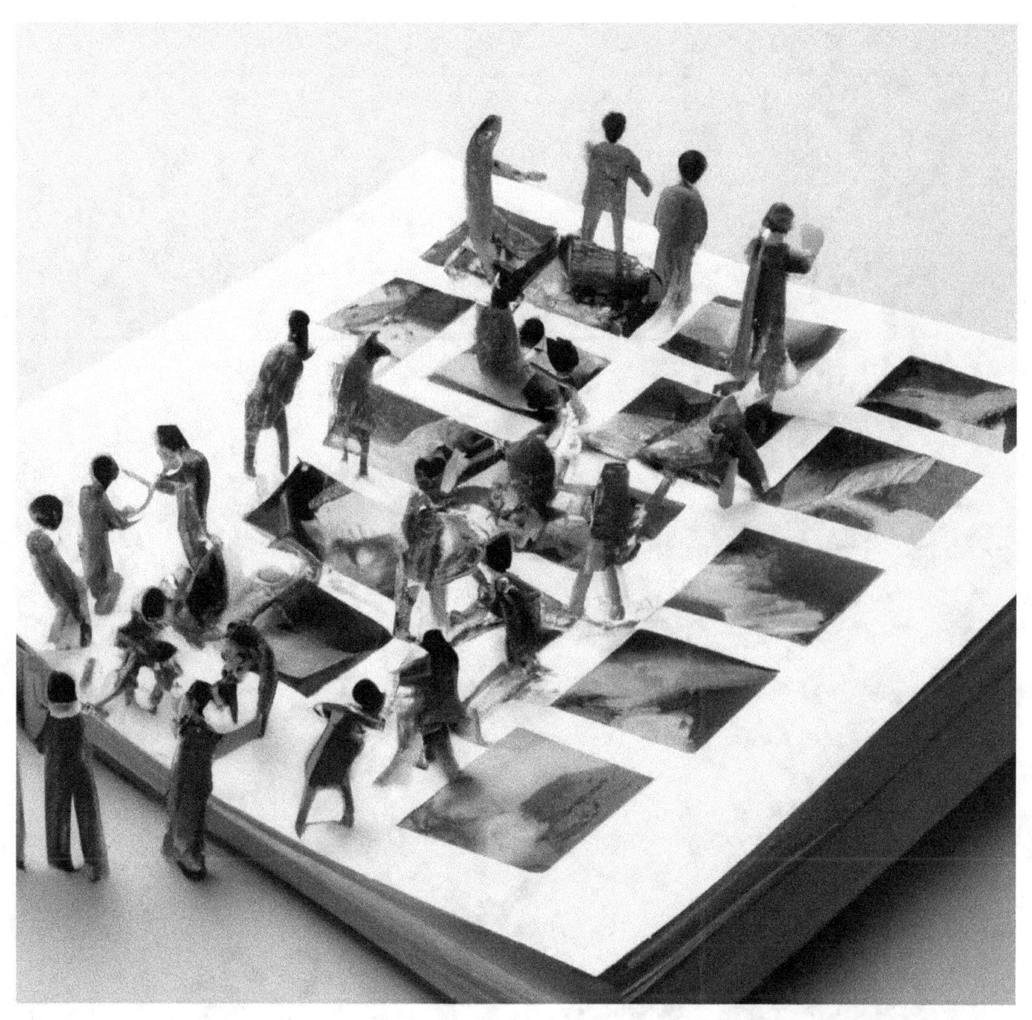

Conclusion

Social life is amazing! Here are 50 amazing facts to prove it:

1. Social life is the best way to connect with others and make friends.

2. Social life is a great way to learn new things and meet new people.

3. Social life is a great way to stay connected with friends and family.

4. Social life is a great way to have fun and relax.

5. Social life is a great way to connect with like-minded people.

6. Social life is a great way to find new friends and romance.

7. Social life is a great way to stay connected with old friends and family.

8. Social life is a great way to make new friends that share your interests.

9. Social life is a great way to find new romantic interests.

10. Social life is a great way to stay connected with old friends and family that have moved away.

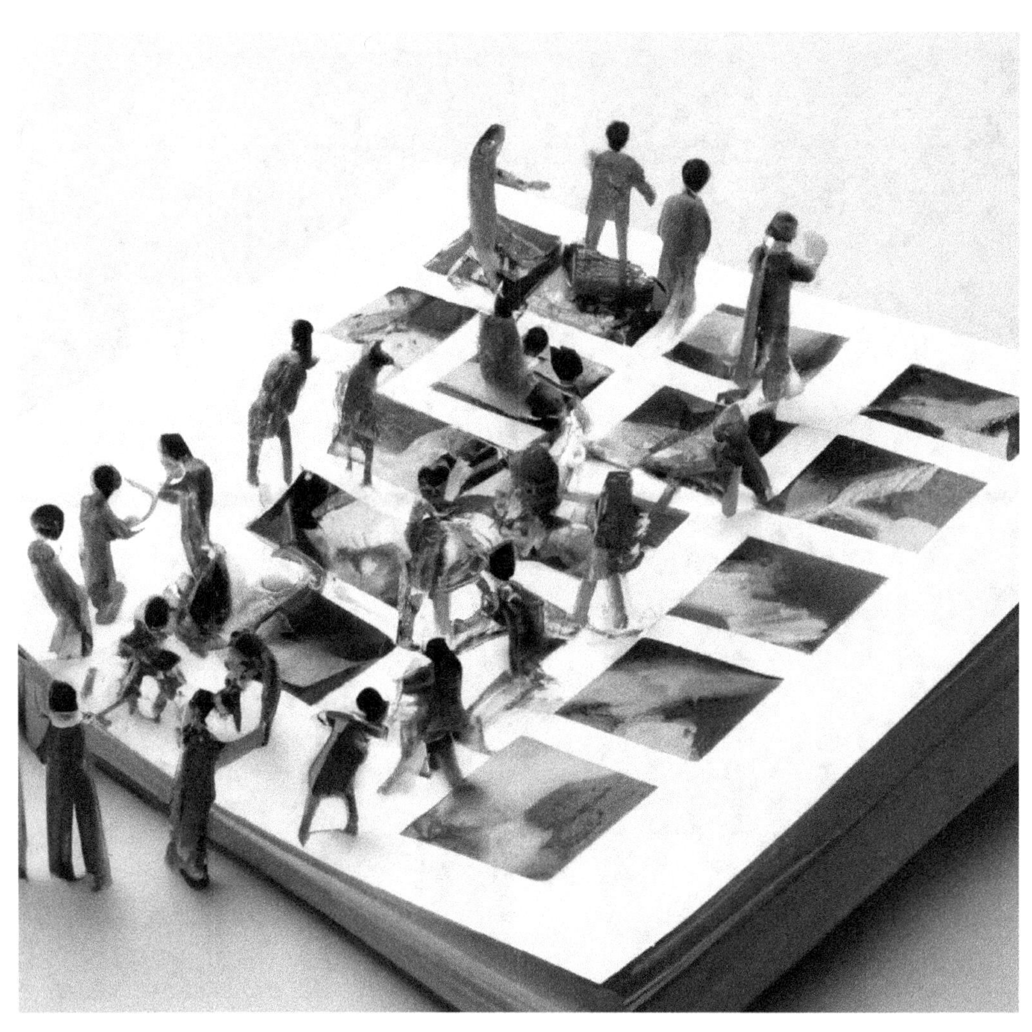

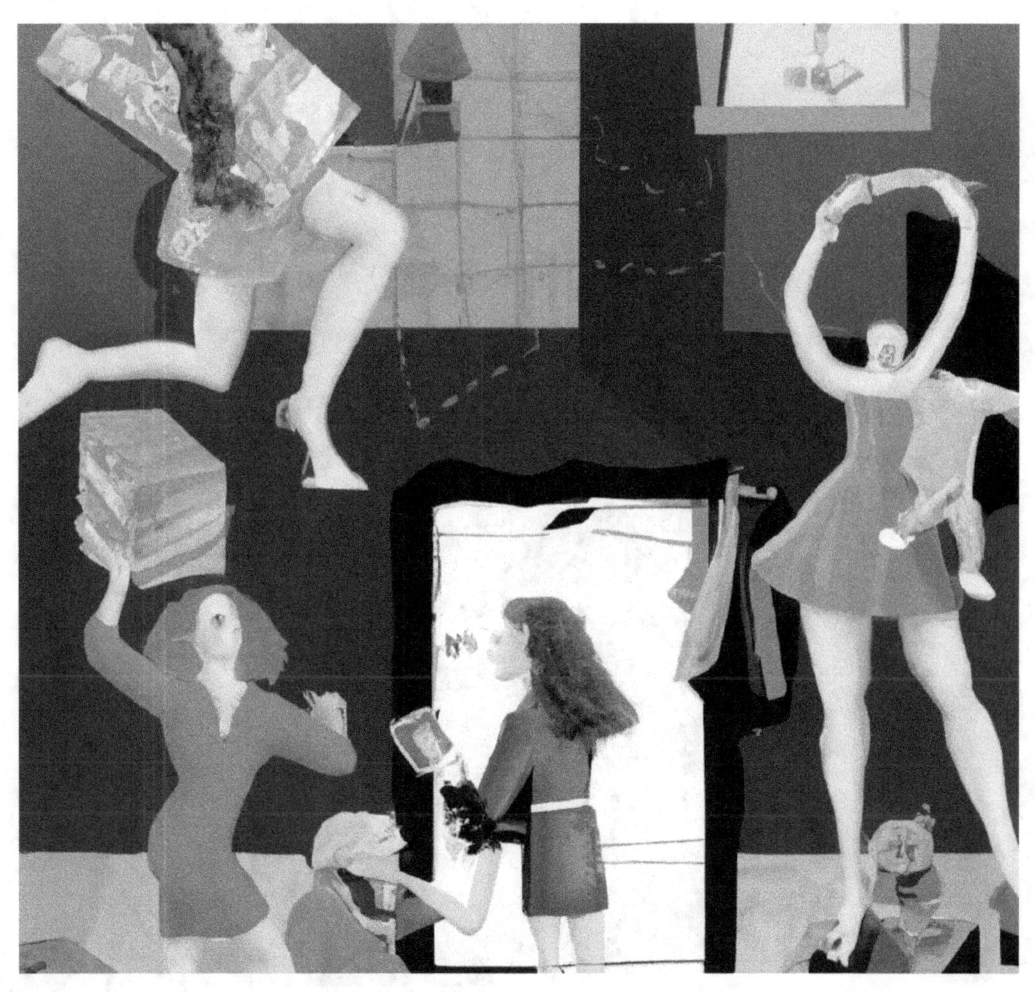

www.ingramcontent.com/pod-product-compliance
Lightning Source LLC
Chambersburg PA
CBHW071555260726
48653CB00008BA/3238